LIVING WITH ULCERATIVE COLITIS

MORE THAN

MEETS
THE EYE

LIAM ROBERTSON

First paperback edition March 2020

Book design by Petya Tsankova
Edited by Ben Way

ISBN 978-1-83853-233-8 (paperback)
ISBN 978-1-83853-234-5 (ebook)

For more information contact:
morethanmeetstheeyebook@gmail.com

FOREWORD

Learning the Hard Way

I suppose sometimes in life it's easy to take things for granted. To get lost in your own world. I mean, why shouldn't you? It's your life after all. You just float along, wrapped up in a tight cocoon of self-importance and a belief in your own superiority, aiming to please yourself each and every day. Although it sounds negative, I believe it's actually a good thing in many ways. It is what drives us to do better, to succeed, to win and to enhance our lives in some way or another. I imagine this selfishness is what has driven many, if not all, the most successful people we know or have heard of throughout history. Now if you are anything like me, you'll probably be guilty of this too from time to time. And if you haven't noticed it before, then you are probably more tightly wrapped up in that cocoon than you realise. Regardless of that, I would like to think you will probably be able to relate to this pretty well.

When I was growing up, maybe not as much a child, but certainly as an early teenager from the ages of 14 and up, I remember feeling an enormous pressure to look or be a certain way. Society tells us that we must have good skin and perfect teeth. We must go to the gym regularly and eat healthy meals, as obviously body fat is a big no-no. We must have the latest brand name plastered across our T-shirts and on-trend trainers. And if you don't, then you should be embarrassed and banished to the realms of the un-cool or socially awkward. Sound familiar? Well, I think that at least for me these pressures got even worse as I grew older. I can remember quite distinctly as I entered my late teens and early twenties these societal demands grew stronger, drastically more expensive and quite frankly much harder to achieve. It went from clothes, trainers and the type of music I chose to listen to, to cars, property and luxury holidays. There was a sudden shame placed upon still living at home with your parents or being unable to drive or not owning a car or whether or not you can afford to go to Ibiza and buy €15 bottles of water.

I feel as the years went on the momentous rise in social media had a massive effect on this. If I were to say most people I know spend almost all day on social media, I would probably be understating the issue. In fact in the first 20 minutes of writing this opening few paragraphs I have already checked my phone three times. The problem is that it can cause us to disconnect from the people and events around us and consistently creates perceptions of what life should be like or how it is for other people and it makes us obsessed about material things. Again, similar to our naturally selfish desires it is not necessarily a bad thing. If it inspires you to train harder or work harder or educate yourself more, then I am all for it. However, there is a fine line between a hunger for more and an underappreciation of what you already have or what's really needed. The problem is most people only learn this the hard way and I was unfortunate enough to be one of them.

At around the age of 21 I started getting quite ill. It mostly consisted of really strong stomach cramps and quite severe bloating. This led to multiple visits to the doctor and hospital on a regular basis. Then at the prime age of 24 years old after two or three years of progressively feeling unwell, my problems finally came to a head and my world was turned upside down. I was diagnosed with ulcerative colitis. If you have never heard of this condition before don't worry because neither had I. I spent a lot of time researching the disease and educated myself as much as I could. My only problem was that most of the information I read online was based on medical facts. Although there are forums where people can speak about their condition, I never really found anything that truly told the story of what it was like to live with this horrible condition. Suddenly all of my material desires faded away. Everything I used to believe about life changed. I quickly realised just how little importance anything in life has if you haven't got your health.

I decided to write this book to share my experience and to give hope to anybody else going through this or something similar – there is a light at the end of the tunnel. This is the story of my journey through sickness, diagnosis and treatment to a new-found wisdom and understanding of life that I will otherwise never have experienced, from my lowest point all the way to where I am today. There is always more than meets the eye.

TABLE OF CONTENTS

ONE

More Than You Bargained For

I'm a pretty normal guy. Or at least I think so. I left school not long before my 16th birthday and went to college. Having played guitar from a young age it was one of my main hobbies growing up and I had decided that a course in music was what I wanted to pursue. However, after a year I realised it wasn't for me. So I left and I worked in a few random jobs before finding an apprenticeship with a large oil and gas service company. Then after a few years I started working offshore on oil rigs in the North Sea. The job was great, paid well and it really was the start of a lifetime career for me. I had finally found something I enjoyed.

It was also around this time that I really started taking training and dieting seriously. This would include a run most mornings, followed by a weight-lifting session in the afternoon and then at least three times a week I would go to a Thai boxing class in the evening too. I would swig on protein shakes morning till night and cut carbs out of almost every meal. If I ate something unhealthy or that I knew wasn't right for me, the guilt that I experienced was indescribable. I would then go out of my way to put in that extra mile in training to make sure I burned it off, as the risk of appearing fat or out of shape wasn't worth the few moments of joy that food would give me. So with my job and my determination in the gym, I was finally overcoming those self-imposed pressures and life was good. I was making great money and I enjoyed my time off. I felt fit and healthy on the inside and out. I really couldn't have asked for anything more.

Then around the age of 21 I went on holiday in the south of Spain. It was a great break – I ate lots of nice food, drank lots of beer and cocktails and soaked up the sun. The day after I got home I was sitting in my living room watching TV, very chilled but with some mild post-holiday blues. All of a sudden my stomach began to churn, but only for a few seconds and then it stopped. My first thought was about the protein shake I had just drunk. I immediately dived off the chair in the direction of the kitchen. Was the protein powder off? I hadn't eaten anything else, so it must have been that, right? But before I could even reach the kitchen doorway another cramp took hold of me. This time it was strong with an almost twisting feeling in my gut. It stopped me in my tracks and in all honesty I panicked for a moment. I stood just at the edge of the doorway and with my hand clamped over my stomach I realised it felt quite hard and tight.

I took another step into the kitchen and then a pain unlike any I had ever experienced before shot through my stomach. It was so strong that my legs gave way and I had to hold onto the side of the cupboard for support. This time it didn't just go away. It sort of faded slightly and my stomach bloated hard and round like a basketball. An overwhelming urge for the toilet came over me. I quickly ran to the bathroom and sat down. I won't go into graphic details, but it was mostly blood and from what I can remember the pain went away almost instantly. However, unbeknown to me this was just the beginning.

I called the doctor first thing in the morning and got an emergency appointment. I explained my symptoms and he said it sounded like a 'dodgy tummy' from some foreign alcohol or meal I had ingested in Spain. I wasn't overly pleased with his diagnosis, but I decided to wait it out nonetheless. At this point, it's worth mentioning that I was feeling absolutely fine. I had woken up that morning like nothing had happened. I even went to the gym and put myself through a pretty gruelling weights session and I didn't feel any different whatsoever. So I suppose it was my fault for maybe not being honest enough about how much pain I had actually been in.

I have always had an issue when visiting doctors while growing up. It's as if the moment you step foot through the surgery door your symptoms magically disappear. I remember one time in particular when I had what I believed to be a chest infection. I had been coughing continuously for days and days. I couldn't sleep and I couldn't even eat properly because I was literally coughing all the time. After a couple of days of this I phoned my doctor to get an appointment, but being such a busy place they didn't have anything available. They told me to try again in the morning, so I did and I was told the same thing. But by this point I was on day four of no real sleep and I couldn't handle it anymore so I argued and argued on the phone, almost exaggerating my symptoms just so I could get an emergency appointment. Finally after almost an hour talking to various people or being put on hold I eventually got one. So I walked up to the surgery coughing and spluttering all the way there. My eyes were bloodshot and saliva sprayed down my T-shirt from coughing so hysterically. I was quite late getting into the waiting room and as soon as I did my name was called. I walked into the room and the doctor told me to take a seat.

The moment I sat down, something happened and I can't explain what it was, although it's happened to me on multiple occasions since then. It was like magic. My cough stopped, my itchy throat disappeared and even the swelling of the glands in my neck seemed to calm down. The doctor asked me what was wrong and that the receptionist had told her I was in a lot of pain. I tried to explain how bad my cough had been, but I could tell by the look on her face that she wasn't taking me seriously. The more I tried to convince her, I could feel my face glowing red with embarrassment as if I was lying. It actually got to the point where I began fake coughing just so I sounded more genuine. Thankfully on this occasion she prescribed me with antibiotics and sent me on my way. It's not always that easy.

By now, almost two full days had passed since my 'dodgy tummy' diagnosis and I was feeling well again. Maybe there was nothing much wrong with me. I woke up the next morning, the alarm beeping loudly at 5:30 am. Although I was on my time off from work, I enjoyed getting up and running in the mornings when it was still dark outside. I had on some old joggers on and the Rocky movie soundtrack blasting through my earphones. It was my favourite time of the day. The run wasn't far, just a loop of around two or three miles, but it was enough to keep me fit and feeling good. It was a great start to the day in my view. On this particular morning I was just finishing the run and was about 50 metres from my front door when the pain in my stomach came on again. The churn was mild and at first I questioned myself on whether it was a stitch from the run or not. I mean, I was breathing quite heavily and struggled near the end so it very well could have been. Then I felt it again, but this time strong and very familiar as the cramps from a couple of days previously. I continued walking and just as I reached my front door a big spasm came on, putting me on my knees and quite embarrassingly causing me to fall headfirst into the door. I remember being glad it was still early and dark.

I quickly rushed inside to the bathroom. It was the same as before. Surely this can't still be a bug from Spain? Or is it? A million worries crossed my mind and although on hindsight this may sound ridiculous, the question did occur to me... am I dying? While sitting on the toilet I decided to Google the symptoms (something you should probably never do for a number of reasons, as it's more likely to put the fear of God in you rather than get an accurate diagnosis) and predictably a lot of the search results were things like bowel cancer and tumours and imminent death. I think it's easy from the outside looking in to tell someone that their thoughts or worries are absurd, but the fact of the matter is when you are in pain and panicking it's very hard not to believe it's serious or that you won't die from it. When the feeling receded I decided that I was going to have a relaxed day in front of the TV and hopefully the rest would do me good.

The day was largely uneventful and as the night drew in I felt the symptoms return. If I couldn't make my mind up whether or not it was serious before, I was certainly sure after this. It was around 8:30 pm in the evening and out of nowhere a mild cramp came on. I bolted straight up and mentally prepared myself for what I knew was about to come. It was almost timed to perfection, around 30 seconds between the first cramp and the second, then about a minute between the second and third. This time I was prepared. As soon as I felt the first one I went straight to the bathroom as I knew a bowel movement was imminent (something I had to learn to do a lot living with colitis, but I will speak about that later), only this time it was different. I stood up thinking it was over and then it hit me again: a strong powerful cramp. Then around 30 seconds later another happened. Then they began to spread further apart, but each lasted longer. They started at a few seconds duration but were now lasting up to 10 seconds or longer. Now when I say the word 'cramp' it might sound reasonably easy to deal with, but these were not normal sensations. These were enormously overwhelming stomach spasms coming from deep inside me. The pain was like nothing I have ever experienced before. It was so strong I began sweating profusely and as each one came on, they got stronger and stronger to the point where I was almost passing out from the pain. Thankfully my partner at the time managed to call the hospital and get advice on what to do.

During the call my condition got increasingly worse and the volume of blood that was coming out of me was terrifying. We requested an ambulance but they told us they couldn't get one to me. Now my partner didn't drive so it was a case of waiting for a taxi, which could have been a long time, or attempt to drive myself. On hindsight I should never have really got in my car that day. I mean I could barely keep my eyes open from the pain, but at the same time I genuinely thought I was going to die and had no choice. At this point the cramps were very similar to what I believe a pregnant woman feels when having contractions while giving birth. They would last for around 10 seconds and then disappear for about a minute or so. So I waited for a break in the cramps and ran out to the car and placed a towel on the seat to avoid getting blood all over the upholstery. I then sat down and started the engine. Just as I did another cramp came on, strong and forceful. I can remember wincing in pain hunched over the steering wheel just praying for it to stop. Then as it faded I put the car into gear and began driving out of the car park and onto the main road. I got a couple of hundred metres up the street when another cramp hit me. I pulled over to the side of the road just as it was coming on and it came on so hard I gripped the wheel in agony, dragging my car closer into the kerb and scraping right down the side of my alloy. I paused for a moment, waiting for it to recede. The second it did I took off again.

The hospital was only about a 20-minute drive away, but on this occasion it took nearly an hour. Although it felt a lot longer to me. It was hands down one of the worst experiences of my life and I hope I never have to experience it again. When I finally arrived I was admitted to a ward and given some strong pain killers and antispasmodic drugs, which really made a difference. If it were not for them I honestly don't think I would have lasted much longer. The pain was just too much. I was so exhausted from the whole ordeal I pretty much fell asleep as soon as my head hit the pillow. The next thing I knew I was awakened by a nurse in the early hours of the morning and she asked if I was okay. I really wish she hadn't because upon waking I found that the painkillers had worn off and the unfortunate realisation of how uncomfortable the bed was really started to sink in. I can remember checking my phone and thinking to myself, okay I'll be out of here in four or five hours. As soon as it's daylight I'll probably be able to go home... Little did I know I was about to spend the next seven days in that bed.

I somehow managed to fall back to sleep, but it was not long before I woke up with a subtle cramping, which I am sure had probably been trying to come on all night, having only been suppressed by the antispasmodic drugs. Thankfully the nurse was in soon after with another dose for me and I was feeling great again in no time. It must have been late in the afternoon before I finally got to speak to a doctor and my expectations of being home before midday were quashed indefinitely. He said he would like to keep me in a little longer for blood tests and to take other samples. In my naivety I translated that to mean I would be home later that evening, but I was again very wrong. When one of the nurses was back to take a blood sample, I innocently asked if I would be late home and she advised me it would be at least a couple of days so they could monitor the condition or at least until the cramps stopped. The problem was they were not stopping. I don't know if it was medication wearing off or my tolerance to it was getting stronger. Or was it that the cramps were actually getting worse? To be honest, I didn't know what to think, but I soon realised that this wasn't going to be a short stopover.

One of the worst aspects of staying in hospital for this kind of investigation and treatment, which is something I didn't get any more comfortable with from the first to the last day, was leaving samples for inspection. The process of emptying your bowels into something that wasn't a toilet was strange enough, but to then put it to one side for someone to come in and inspect after you were done was absolutely horrendous. I know people say not to worry about it and that doctors and nurses see this sort of things all the time, but to me that didn't make it any easier. It was an extremely unpleasant part of hospital life that I also hope I never have to experience again. The next problem was that I had to start on a clear liquid diet, which for someone like myself who was used to having five or six meals a day as a minimum was difficult to say the least. What I would say is that the cramps certainly became milder and almost non-existent after a couple of days of eating like this. Despite this I couldn't help but count all the grams of protein I was missing out on and I was convinced I could see my arms actually decreasing in size throughout the day, especially around the biceps. This certainly didn't make me feel any better and suddenly I had a new reason for getting out sooner: the gym.

I also had to have a slightly uneasy phone call with my boss to tell him why I couldn't go to work. I was due to fly out the next day and there was no sign of me getting out of hospital anytime soon. The conversation didn't go too well and because I still didn't know what was wrong with me he started asking lots of questions about my symptoms, which I really didn't feel comfortable talking about. I mean, what did he want me to say? The reason I can't come to work is because I'm having cramps in my stomach and an undiagnosed bleeding from my rectum? I had only told my parents what was happening at this point. I hadn't even told any of my friends I was in hospital and I certainly wasn't about to go into the details with my boss. Anyway, I think it was the evening of day three that a young-looking doctor accompanied by two even younger-looking student doctors entered my room. He briefly asked how I was feeling and then continued to whisper with the other two while examining the clipboard at the end of my bed.

He then asked if anyone had spoken with me yet and proceeded to tell me his thoughts on my condition. He said that I had come down with a case of gastroenteritis. If you are reading this and don't know what that is, then let me give you a brief explanation. It is a reasonably common condition that can affect men and women of all ages that causes diarrhoea, vomiting and abdominal pain. It usually comes from some sort of viral or bacterial infection. All in all it's pretty much a bad stomach bug that lasts for around a week. Unfortunately for me this particular bug was viral and therefore there wasn't any medication I could take to solve the problem. It was just a case of waiting it out. So it turns out the 'dodgy tummy' diagnosis maybe wasn't all that wrong after all. Although slightly underestimated, it was good to find out that it was indeed a tummy bug. Anyway, after another few days of being on a drip and having my blood tested I was finally allowed to go home. I may have slightly downplayed how I was feeling, but I had been there almost a full week and I really wanted to leave. I was discharged with a big box of medication, mostly antispasmodic tablets and painkillers, and sent on my way. I was out, I was free and it was finally over. Or at least I thought it was. And by rights it should have been after everything I had been through in hospital. It should have been all over. However, nobody could have ever foreseen what was to happen next.

My life was about to change for ever.

TWO

There's Nothing Wrong with You

Before you read this chapter please understand that it is not a criticism of anyone in the National Health Service nor is it anything negative about any of the treatment I have received. This is just an honest recollection of my experience during this time.

After leaving hospital and having had nothing except liquids for several days, to say I was hungry and craving bad food was an understatement. I was starving, and for the first time in my life using that statement was actually true. My mouth was watering on the way home in the car at just the mere thought of a burger or chips or chocolate. In fact what I craved most was toast and butter – specifically brown seeded bread covered with a large scraping of Lurpak. I like to leave the toast to cool down a bit before I spread it. Saves the butter melting and keeps it thick. There was an art to this. And I was at a point in my life where I would usually only allow myself bread as a special treat on a weekend, so the mastery of this art was very important to me. It had to be perfect.

Needless to say, this was the first thing I did upon arriving home. Not one, not two, not three but four slices of a beautiful brown granary seeded loaf and a large slab of lightly salted butter carefully slicked across the surface of each. It was absolutely heavenly. Although even in this heightened state of hunger and cravings, I really did struggle to finish them all. My stomach must have shrunk dramatically over the week in hospital with next to no food and the effects of it were very noticeable. I did however manage to finish them with the support of a giant mug of tea. It was good to be home, but I would say that this was probably as good as things were going to get over the next couple of weeks. I can remember even later that night feeling a little pain in my stomach. I put it down to the reintroduction of solid foods again, especially the little seeds on the bread as they were so hard and could be difficult to digest.

I woke up the next day feeling reasonably well. I still had a craving for a burger and chips, so at lunchtime I got into the car and drove to a drive-thru not far from my house. I ordered an XL burger and chips and a milkshake. It tasted even better than I had imagined and thankfully the toast and other things I had eaten the day before had obviously helped stretch my stomach a bit. I devoured the burger and fries so quickly I actually almost forgot I had eaten it. By the time I arrived home I could tell something wasn't right though. I couldn't put my finger on exactly what it was, but I knew it wasn't good. Later that night I woke up with my stomach bloated and sore. It wasn't cramps like before, but just a dull pain and bloating. I went to the toilet and there it was again: blood. I was a little confused as to whether it was the remainder of the gastroenteritis or if it was something more sinister. I tried to continue as normal for the next day or two in the hope it would go away but it didn't really get any better. Constant bloating and constant pain. I decided to go speak to my doctor again and get advice on what to do. Luckily I got an emergency appointment for later that day and when I walked into the room explained that I had just got out of hospital after a case of viral gastroenteritis. The first question she asked me, and it's something I will never ever forget, was: "Did you follow the diet plan?" I thought to myself, what diet plan? I hadn't been given one. In fact I can distinctly remember having a conversation with the nurse before I left regarding my cravings for a burger and chips and her reply was something about how good stodgy food is upon leaving hospital.

I had to pause for a moment before answering the GP. I had mixed emotions. Part of me was angry and frustrated that I was allowed to just walk out of hospital without any guidance or medical advice on what to do or not do, but part of me was also a little embarrassed because when she said it, it did very much make a lot of sense. I mean, coming home after a seven-day stomach illness and going out for a burger and chips surely can't be good for you. I suppose at the time I was so tired and hungry I wasn't really thinking logically. So I told her that I hadn't been given a diet plan and that I had a burger. The doctor actually laughed as if I was joking, but then immediately realised from the look on my face that I wasn't. She was concerned, which in turn made me very concerned. Anyway, following that conversation she provided me with a list of food that I could and couldn't eat and gave advice about reintroducing other food back into your diet. Although I was pretty sure it was too late and the damage was already done, I decided to stick to the list anyway. Just in case. Unfortunately for me, things didn't really get any better. In fact they got worse. A lot worse.

The bloating in my stomach by this point was pretty constant, although on a pain level it was reasonably manageable. I was facing two by-products of the bloating. First was a large increase in bowel movement frequency, or at least a sense of urgency to go, and the second was the pressure it placed upon my bladder, making it harder to retain urine for long periods of time. This made life very difficult for me and I really struggled to adjust. One of the biggest problems I had was returning to work and it really was one of the hardest things I have ever had to do. In my job working away from home, having to share rooms with people as well as bathrooms, you can imagine how someone needing to use the toilet 10 times a day didn't make for an easy life. And if I am being honest I was embarrassed about it. I used to sit and wonder if people were counting how many times I would go in. I can remember one day we were in the middle of a job and I said to my supervisor that I needed to go to the bathroom. He says "Again? You're never out of there. You can't go until we finish this!" I can remember struggling through the last hour of work, my stomach had inflated like a beach ball and it was hard and sore to touch. I could barely walk, let alone move around and pick heavy items up.

At one point I genuinely thought I was going to bleed through my trousers. The bloating was so intense that I couldn't hold it in. I remember checking my watch and there was still over 30 minutes to go before the end of shift. I feel like the stress of this moment actually knocked years off my life. By the time I was allowed to go, I couldn't walk properly. I had to tiptoe all the way back to the locker room to make sure I didn't leak any blood or worse into my clothes. Looking back I still don't know why I didn't just hold my hands up and say I'm sick and I need to go. I was just so career-minded and focused on progressing that I was in a constant battle between looking after my health and staying on top of my work. Not to mention the fact that I had a house and a car and bills to pay. That didn't exactly help the situation. As soon as I got home from work the following week I ended up having to go straight back to hospital. I explained the situation, but they told me it was because of the gastroenteritis and that everything would sort itself out.

Over the next couple of weeks my symptoms gradually became worse. The toilet frequencies were on the increase, the blood was now accompanied by an unexplained mucus, and the external effects it was having on my life really started to gain momentum. When I say that this illness was ruining my life that is no exaggeration. It affected my ability to maintain relationships – I didn't want to go out and socialise with people, I stopped going to the gym as much, I became stressed and depressed and all of these factors are all linked to each other in a vicious circle. My life began collapsing around me and I couldn't do anything about it. I visited my doctor on a regular basis, sometimes more than once a week. Each time the symptoms got worse, I would call and get an appointment and tell them about it and each time I would be given a blood test and sent home. They said nothing was wrong with me over and over and over again. I finally convinced them that I needed a referral and I was booked in for a colonoscopy. For the people who haven't experienced this procedure I will briefly explain. It is basically a camera on the end of a flexible cable that is inserted into your rectum and then fed up through your colon. The view from the camera is fed live to a screen where the doctors and nurses will examine the condition of your colon. At this point I didn't have a clue what it would be like, I was just happy there was some progress being made. Unfortunately the appointment was still a couple of months away and I had to try to struggle on.

My condition got worse with every passing day. Sometimes I would feel vaguely okay and think to myself, am I on the mend here? Is it going away? Then I would wake up the next day twice as bad as I was before. During this time I kept a lot of it to myself. I didn't really say much to my friends or the people around me. Life became quite difficult because everywhere I went had to revolve around access to a toilet. When I was going out I always had to think about where the closest public toilets were, or if it was a restaurant or bar would the toilets be open or would there be more than one. There is nothing more soul-destroying than running to the bathroom when you urgently need to go and to find it out of action or closed for cleaning or for someone to already be using it. Things like the theatre or concerts were impossible for me, as the huge queues and wait times just made it too risky for me. Most nightclubs were also off-limits because of the terrible state of the facilities and lack of toilet paper in most of them. The best way I used to explain it to people was about the sensation of needing to go. There was no 'holding it in' or 'waiting until later.' When I had to go, I meant it. It was like, 'right now, I have 30 seconds to find a bathroom.' When I was having a bad day, life was just easier if I stayed at home. If I'm being completely honest this was more frequent than not.

Finally the week of the colonoscopy arrived. I was

absolutely exhausted. I hadn't been sleeping well at all because of the bloating and pain during the night and this had really started to take its toll. I had just come home from work after two weeks of night shift and there was a package waiting for me that had been sent through the post. I opened it up to find a letter and some booklets with information on the colonoscopy procedure. There was also a packet of laxative sachets. You had to drink those 24 hours before going into hospital and then fast with only water and one or two other things allowed. The purpose of it was to ensure your bowel was empty so the camera could see everything it needed to see. This particular laxative was called Picolax and I believe it was a blackcurrant flavour. It was absolutely vile and I really struggled to get it down. Eventually I did and it wasn't long before it started to take effect. The laxative effect is like nothing I have ever experienced before in my life. It was just constant, all day and all night. I actually had to use the bathroom while sitting in the hospital waiting room and started to panic. What if I need to go when the camera is in? What if it, you know, comes out? Again, people say doctors and nurses see this stuff all the time, but like I said before this does not make it any easier for me.

I entered a changing room and stripped off all my clothes. I then put on a gown and filled out some paperwork. I was led into another room and lay down on a bed. I immediately did not feel comfortable at all. I thought, perhaps quite naively, that it was going to be a doctor and possibly a nurse in the room. The camera would be inserted discreetly and it would be all over and done within a few minutes. That was not the case at all. There were six or seven people in the room in total. From what I can remember, there was a specialist, two junior doctors, two nurses and a student. This was all a little intimidating for me, considering I was pretty much naked and when laid on the bed really had no way of hiding my privates due to the cut and length of the gown. I think what also didn't help was that most of the people in the room were quite young, roughly around my age or possibly younger. This for some reason made me even more nervous. Things started running through my head like, do I know them? Do they know me? Do they know people I know? In hindsight that's not important at all, but at the time – and on top of everything else – it made it really difficult for me to relax. That feeling didn't last long though. All those worries, fears, nerves and anxieties disappeared and I can tell you why in one word: sedation. I believe it's a combination of different drugs you are given and I can't remember what they're called. However, it was absolutely incredible.

A few moments later I did not feel anything. I was drowsy, but all the worries were gone. I began chatting away and making conversation with everyone in the room. It was great. After a few moments I was asked to lie on my side and try to relax. They guided me through the whole procedure as it was happening. This is another aspect of it that I clearly knew nothing about. I was under the impression that it was going to be a camera just placed inside me, maybe by a few inches. I didn't realise that it gets fed right through your entire colon. It is actually quite amazing how it's done. I would say the camera insertion itself was reasonably painless, more just uncomfortable. The real pain or at least major discomfort comes from the air. They pump this into you so that your colon expands and they can manoeuvre the camera better and see more detail. It is without a doubt the worst part of the whole procedure and I could not have managed it without the sedation, although I have read about people who have done it without and I take my hat off to them. That is no mean feat.

The examination continued and I was sort of floating in and out of consciousness. I watched the camera footage on the screen as much as I could, but to be honest I couldn't really see anything. Unfortunately for me it turns out they couldn't either. The procedure ended and I was taken through to another room to sleep off the effects of the sedation and wait for someone to come pick me up and take me home. When I woke up they told me the bad news: the results were inconclusive. They couldn't see as clearly as they hoped and the parts they could see looked absolutely fine. I was back to square one.

The following few months were even harder than the ones before. I got the feeling that I was starting to annoy the doctors I was speaking to because in their minds there was nothing wrong with me. When I used to call up and ask for an appointment it was almost always a different doctor I would see each time. I remember on one particular occasion I had seen the same doctor two or three times in a row. I was complaining that I still wasn't feeling well and told him about the bloating and soreness. Then during another visit where I was almost breaking down I asked him if he thought it was normal to be constantly bloated and bleeding from your rectum up to 10 times a day. He proceeded to tell me that my colonoscopy showed nothing sinister, my blood tests had come back fine and that there was nothing wrong with me. I will never forget his closing words. He said, "What do you want me to do?" I can remember feeling very confused and lost. I was in a pretty bad state of mind at the time. My life had been turned upside down, I was in pain, had become unfit and unhealthy, lost touch with a lot of friends and the only person in my mind who could fix the problem didn't seem all that enthusiastic about fixing it. I was in a very bad place.

THREE

I Have Bad News for You

A month or so later I was finally referred to a private specialist in gastroenterology. I sat with him and explained all of my symptoms. He immediately said it is one of two things – I either have irritable bowel syndrome (IBS) or a form of inflammatory bowel disease (IBD). At the time these acronyms were already familiar to me because I had seen them come up on forums and webpages during research of my symptoms. IBS had also been mentioned by my doctor a few times as a possible cause. He told me that it was a little harder to treat, but it can be pretty much cured eventually. However, IBD was more straightforward to treat, but it was a chronic disease with worse symptoms. He said he hoped it was IBS and we could get it fixed. I found great comfort in his expertise and I immediately started seeing light at the end of the tunnel.

My specialist booked me in for another colonoscopy

and within a few weeks I was ready. This time I was not so nervous and actually weirdly a little excited. I felt like I was making rapid progress in my search for an answer to my problem and I was at the last hurdle before getting well again. The process was pretty much the same as before. Different location and different people, but the equipment and procedure was pretty much identical. The only difference was this time I had a private room to myself, but to be honest the sedative is so strong that you probably wouldn't notice either way. So the camera went up, he checked everything he needed to check and I was wheeled back to my room to recover. I can't quite remember how long it was before he came into the room, but it felt like no time at all. He sat down and said, "I'm sorry but I have bad news. You have ulcerative colitis."

It is quite a surreal experience for a doctor to inform you that you have a disease that you have never even heard of before. I mean, I maybe had heard about the condition at some point in my life, but in my selfish cocoon I had never taken the time to really understand it. In fact, other than cancer purely due to its infamy, I had never really taken an interest or sought out knowledge of any illness – diabetes, kidney failure, gout, you name it – that did not directly affect me. And even now with hindsight, why should I? There are already enough things in life that affect me that I don't understand or have the time to study, never mind all the things that don't. When he actually told me the bad news, I was keener for him to get out of the room so I could Google the condition and read about it rather than actually sit and hear him out. I very naively convinced myself – with no justifiable reason – that it would not be a big deal and that I would be able to fix it or at the very least there would be some magical solution that would make it all go away. Little did I know that chronic illnesses do not ever really go away. Up until this point in my life I thought the word 'chronic' was a term to describe the severity of a condition or symptoms rather than its persistence. And now when I read its definition in the dictionary as 'constantly recurring' I couldn't agree with it more – especially in relation to ulcerative colitis.

One thing that had never really crossed my mind at the time was to ask why. Why me? What had I done to be struck down with such a horrible disease? I think some point later I began to question the poor decisions I had made in my life and feared it was some sort of supreme form of karma coming back to bite me as retribution for all my sins. I was later to realise that in fact it was quite the opposite. There are no clear-cut reasons as to why people actually get ulcerative colitis. However, research has now suggested there are a number of aggravating factors that include diet and stress. In my case, I had a family history of bowel and colon problems so it was pretty much put down to my genetics as opposed to something I did or how I lived my life.

So I eventually got home and first thing the next morning went to my doctor to pick up a prescription.

'Pentasa' it said on the box, '2g twice a day.' It was a nonsteroidal anti-inflammatory drug (NSAID) and I was super excited to take it and hopeful that it was going to help me. My walk to the pharmacy pretty much became a run. Then as soon as I got home I hadn't even got my jacket off before I had the first dose swallowed. They were big chunky tablets, 4 of them at a time, and if you didn't swallow them quickly they began to dissolve in your mouth. Five minutes passed by and I wasn't feeling any better. Is that not how this works? I know it sounds crazy, but I genuinely believed that I was going to start feeling better straight away. A day passed, a week and then a month. My condition wasn't even stabilising, never mind getting better. I would say I was just as bad, probably actually worse, than what I was when I first started taking them. They had no effect on me whatsoever. There were one or two days around this time that I could barely get out of bed because my stomach was so sore and bloated. I went back to see my doctor and explained that the Pentasa was really not working and that I was actually feeling worse. He immediately suggested I try a course of steroids called Prednisone. These tablets were one of the best and worst things that ever happened to me in relation to my condition and mental state and I will explain why.

The course was eight weeks with a steady decline in the treatment. So you start on 40mg a day for a week and then reduce it by 5mg a week for eight weeks. I got the prescription and picked the tablets up. As you can imagine I wasn't holding my breath. This had been going on for around four years now since I originally got ill and I was still suffering even worse than I ever was. I took the tablets and continued with my day. Later that evening I was cooking some food and looked at the clock on my kitchen wall and seen it said 7:00 pm. I then realised I hadn't been to the toilet since lunchtime and I hadn't needed to. I actually panicked for a moment and thought, is something wrong with me? And then I remembered the tablets. Surely not? Am I cured? I felt like doing a backflip across the kitchen table I was so happy. I went to bed that night and had the first full night of sleep I can remember for ages. I did wake up quite early, maybe around 5:00 am, but I had slept right through to that point. No toilet breaks, no bloating, no pain. Just pure, deep sleep.

I woke up refreshed, tidied the house, went to the gym and had two meals before I needed the bathroom. And even when I did, that was the last of it for the day. There was still a tiny bit of blood, but it had almost gone and by day three or four it had completely disappeared. The Prednisone did something else to me too and I still can't explain exactly what it was, but it was like a stimulus for my brain. A bit like a subtle version of the super brain tablets from the movie Limitless. If you haven't seen it, it's basically about Bradley Cooper who takes an experimental drug called NZT-48 that makes him super focused and smart and efficient. In the film it goes to quite extreme lengths, which obviously didn't happen to me, but in a very mild way that is exactly what they did to me. I don't know if it was the relief of my symptoms or the tablets themselves, but I was so happy and focused. Everything in my life was flowing well. I was getting up and running again, I was lifting weights again, my social life had started to pick up because I had gained confidence about going out to places again. Life was great and to be honest I thought this was how it was going to be for me going forward. It didn't quite turn out like that. I ended the eight-week course and still felt great. I must have been around a week after when I was sleeping one night and I woke up with my stomach feeling quite tight and sore. I went to the toilet and there it was, like a knife straight to the heart – blood everywhere.

Over the next week or so I just got worse and worse until I was at the point I was when first diagnosed. It absolutely destroyed me. I could have cried. And actually I think I did once or twice around this time. I was mentally and physically exhausted and had no energy left to deal with it. I remember one of my friends who was a sergeant in the military for a number of years used to tell me about techniques hostage takers would use to get information out of people. One of them was to allow the hostage to be set loose and tell them they are free to go. They would obviously start running away, overwhelmed with joy thinking it was all over, but the hostage takers would have someone waiting a couple of miles away at the end of the road and as soon as the person got close they would just grab them and take them back. The feeling of being free and then getting locked up again would demoralise them so much that they would just give up and confess everything they knew. That's how I felt after the steroids. It was like I had finally been freed from this torture that had been holding me down for the last few years and then coming off them was just like the hostage takers grabbing me again and locking me back up. I fell into a depression and really just had given up. I think if it wasn't for my being able to keep my job and certain few positive people around me I would have never got through this time.

I eventually got back to see my specialist and he suggested I move up to a stronger drug. This time it was an immunosuppressant to suppress the body's immune system. The idea that ulcerative colitis was an autoimmune disease – i.e. one where the body attacks and damages its own tissues – meant that by suppressing the immune system the colitis would also be suppressed. However, this did come with some major risks of its own as you can imagine. One was the increased risk in lymphoma, which is cancer of the lymph glands, as well as some other types of skin cancer. I was hesitant at first and provisionally agreed with his suggestion. He thought it would be best if I went away offshore and got my work done, then we would start on the course as soon as I got back so I had a couple of weeks at home to ensure any nasty side effects would be cleared or at least identified before I went away again and allow us to monitor my blood. However, as I left his room and began the drive home I had decided it wasn't for me. Although in terms of medical risk it was reasonably low, I still felt very uneasy about it and thought that there must be something else I could try.

I was due to go away to work that week and my stomach had been hurting really badly in the days leading up to it. Although I had made my mind up that taking the tablets was too high a risk, the bloating and long hours each day spent sitting on the toilet had begun to really sway my feeling about it. Going offshore for that trip gave me the opportunity to think about it all and decide what I really wanted to do. I spent the next three weeks researching almost every forum I could find about the drug, which was typically prescribed to prevent organ rejection after a transplant, which was a fact that I found so odd and so unrelated to my condition. It certainly didn't make me feel any better about it, but I kept reading regardless. The drug is called Azathioprine and there were hundreds and hundreds of posts on both official and non-official forums about people's views and experiences of it. I read them all. Twice. My condition had worsened again while I was away at work and some days I needed to go to the bathroom up to 20 times. It was completely impractical and made my job impossible to do. I felt like I was at rock bottom. My quality of life at this point was so poor I genuinely asked myself the question, would taking these tablets and somehow being unlucky enough to get cancer or some other serious illness be that bad? I was in a place where I was close to giving up my job and close to losing my friends, so I made the decision that I was just going to take them and hope for the best.

I started taking Azathioprine. I believe it was 100mg a day. My specialist told me it would take around two or three months to begin working. At this point even two or three minutes would have been too long, never mind months. I started taking the tablets and crossed my fingers, although if I am honest I did not have any faith in it working at all. Part of this course was getting weekly blood tests to make sure my liver function wasn't affected and that my blood count was okay, so a week later I went for my first test. I received a call from the doctor within about two days asking me to come in and speak to them regarding the results. I knew straight away that this was not going to be good news. I went to see him and he asked how I was feeling. I said I felt terrible, but that wasn't anything new. He then went on to tell me blood cell count wasn't normal and I may be anaemic. It could have been down to the new tablets or it could have been due to my continual loss of blood from the colitis. Either way it wasn't a great place to be. Unfortunately there wasn't much that could be done about it. We just had to monitor it and see how it went, and if it got really bad we could maybe look at stopping the Azathioprine. I thought, great another stumbling block and something new stopping me from getting better. It's just one thing after another. He also gave me a prescription for some iron tablets that were meant to help but didn't. So again, being quite naive I had no real knowledge of what it meant to be anaemic either, but I was soon to find out.

I had begun working in the office for a while to try get my condition back on track because being away and trying to get to the bathroom 20 times a day was just absolutely impossible. I can remember days when I would struggle to keep my eyes open at my desk and just wanted to fall asleep. People would say, you're looking tired, did you not get a good night's sleep? I would think to myself, yes I slept well (or as well as you can with colitis). It turns out it was to do with the anaemia because as soon as my blood cell count eventually settled, those tired feelings disappeared. I feel sorry for people who suffer from that on a serious level as I just don't know how they cope.

After a month or two I started getting a little impatient and wanted to get better sooner. I decided there must be more options than just this one linear route of medication. There had to be something I could do. I started researching all of the different theories about diet and juicing, Eastern spiritual healing and even something called faecal transplant (I will get into more detail about these later). I decided to run a few ideas past my specialist, but he immediately warned me against them. He said there wasn't enough medical proof that any of these actually worked and he didn't want it to disrupt the effect of the Azathioprine. I thought to myself, the effect of the Azathioprine? I have been taking it for two months and it hadn't done a damn thing anyway. I did feel like telling him that, but instead I politely agreed and decided to wait it out. Another month passed and

I still didn't feel any better, in fact just as before I felt worse. When I reached month four and there was still no change, I ended up getting really down. I was in a dark place. I could barely bring myself to go to work, even after transferring to office-based responsibilities, I couldn't socialise and I couldn't maintain a normal life in any way whatsoever. It had put a strain on my relationship with my partner too, which perhaps inevitably led to the end for us. Each of these things placed stress on me and in turn that made my colitis worse, and then more aspects of my life got difficult, which then stressed me even more and so on.

This went round and round and round and I had pretty much given up everything in my life. Although working in the office, I was on sick leave from my real job and therefore reduced wages, which at this point was only just enough to cover my bills, pay for my flat and keep my car on the road. Having money to actually live and do things was out of my reach, even if I wanted to. I split from my partner. I lost touch with the few friends I had and missed out on some major events, including significant birthdays and one of my best friend's wedding. The next couple of months were a bit of blur to be honest and I can't quite pinpoint when but something amazing happened. One day I went to the driving range with one of my friends and hit a few balls. When we got there he suggested we have a round of golf instead, which usually would have been impossible for me because four hours round a course is far too long to be away from toilet access, but for some reason I wasn't even thinking about it and just agreed. We were on hole 11 and just about to tee off. He turned to me and just casually commented that it had been almost a year since we had last played. I said, really – has it been that long? He said yes, so your stomach must be better now? I began to reply saying no and it hit me. I hadn't been to the toilet since that morning and it was now mid-afternoon.

It was one of those light bulb moments. I felt confused. Has the Azathioprine finally started to take effect? How had I made it all day without needing to go? I made it all the way round the course and the drive home without the need for the toilet even crossing my mind. Was I finally healed? It seemed too good to be true. I awoke the next day after a full night's sleep with no bloating and no pain. I decided to push myself and see how it felt. So I pulled on my shorts and hoodie and went out for a run. I kind of expected a bit of a flare up or some pain, but there was nothing. I finished the run and got home fine. I think it was this point here where my mood completely changed. It was if the clouds had finally cleared and the sun was shining. And it was shining bright and warm. Other than the eight-week period when I was on the steroid course, this was the first time in around four or five years that I hadn't been ill. It was one of the most exciting moments of my adult life. I can't remember if it was a line in a song or if I read it in a book somewhere, but the words, 'Sunny days wouldn't be special, if it wasn't for rain. Joy wouldn't feel so good, if it weren't for pain' stuck in my head. It was never truer than it was to me at that exact point in my life. It had only taken six months, but it had finally started to do the job it was supposed to and my symptoms were gone. Now I know reading this it probably sounds stupid, but even just being able to get in my car and drive to the shops for food or something without having to plan it around bathroom breaks or the distance or traffic was absolute bliss. Even a full night's sleep without any bloating or pain was amazing, never mind the big things like getting back into the gym, nights out and even holidays. I got back to work, got a medical done and was finally approved to go offshore as normal. It was great. I spent the next six or seven months really just making up for lost time. Socialising with friends again, playing sports and I even managed to get a few weekends away.

Azathioprine was my new best friend and had restored my faith in the health service. I was officially healed and my life was back on track.

FOUR

Too Good to be True

I find it funny how people, including myself, refer to diseases or illnesses they suffer from for long periods of time as a possession. It is always 'my' colitis, as opposed to colitis on its own as a separate thing. I mean I would never refer to a cold or flu as 'my cold' or 'my flu,' but it seems after some time of suffering you naturally create a bond or connection with an illness and it sort of becomes part of you and who you are. I would say that these types of things, that also include major accidents or trauma, are the most powerful, character-defining forces you will ever experience in life and in some ways I am thankful for it. I think it was this mindset that really got me through the hard times.

So my life was back to normal. I got fit again and got some of my shape back – some, but not much. I started socialising again and re-strengthened some relationships that had broken down when I was ill. I was back doing my normal job and I was making good money again. All in all I was happy and I was healthy thanks to the wonders of Azathioprine. And I think a lot of it was down to the fact I had a new perspective on life. I no longer wanted for material things or felt the need to impress anyone. Success, to me, really just meant staying healthy and fit. I didn't necessarily care about having the best clothes or going on lavish holidays or getting more likes on a social media post. I was just content with not having colitis and having a normal-ish life. It is amazing how these things, although terrible at the time, really make a positive difference to you in the long run. I think I was about six months into remission from my colitis and I can remember waking up from a night out feeling a little unwell. I wasn't sure if it was from the beer the night before or a colitis feeling, but the symptoms were very similar. It really did give me a sharp reminder of just how bad it used to be because I think by this point I'd almost forgotten what it actually felt like.

I wasn't one for going out partying much those days anyway and I only really went out on special occasions. So I made the decision to limit my alcohol consumption and also avoid beer, just in case it was having a bad effect on me. I then concentrated on just getting healthier and fitter for several months and everything was going well. It is worth mentioning that during this period of being well again that I had been eating really healthy meals and been on a strict low carb diet. One of the main parts of this diet was my use of protein shakes to supplement my meals and to keep my macronutrients correct. If you are unsure of why that is important I will explain. It is basically the main categories different foods fall into – carbohydrates, proteins, fats. Typically high protein diets that are low in fats and carbohydrates tend to be the most favoured diets for losing weight quickly while maintaining muscle mass. However, although there is no real clinical proof I now know that these protein powder shakes that so many people drink are nothing but bad news for a variety of reasons, but I will speak about that later. I am going to blame them among some other things as one of the biggest aggravators of my colitis, and unfortunately I found that out all too late. I think I was well into my 10th month of remission by this point, approaching the one-year mark and very happy.

It was a Sunday morning and I was out for a round of golf with my friend. It was a bright blue sky and the sun was absolutely beating down. We had a bacon roll and a coffee before heading out to the course. I completed the full 18 – well, almost. I was on the last hole at the green just about ready to head back to the clubhouse and go home when all of a sudden my stomach cramped up. And when I say cramped up, I mean like a full-on spasm. It almost dropped me to the ground. There was not a single part of me that thought it may have been my colitis coming back. In my head that life had been and gone and was never coming back. Or at least that's what I told myself. I ran to the bathroom and the worst possible thing happened. Blood. Lots and lots of it. More than I can ever remember. And within a split second I was back in that dark place. Was I dying? It may sound like an exaggeration, but that is genuinely what went through my head. I decided to put it down to something I had eaten and that it wasn't my colitis. I was trying to keep positive. I began driving home and within around two minutes of being in the car my stomach just inflated again. It was so bad that I had to pull over. Luckily for me the back road from the golf course was in a forested area where there were no cars and plenty of shelter. So yes I had to do it on the side of the road – not one of my proudest moments, but it also wasn't the first time. I had grown a certain resilience to the worry or embarrassment of having to do this sort of thing. It was part and parcel of having ulcerative colitis. I finally got home and I jumped straight into the shower. I began to get anxious about whether it was something I had eaten or if it was the colitis back with a vengeance. Unfortunately for me it was the latter.

I was in a state of total disbelief. I had been super healthy for months and months. Not even a hint of anything wrong. No blood, no mucus, no cramps, no bloating. Then suddenly at a click of the fingers I was ill again. What did I do wrong? I started racking my brain to think of what I ate or what I did that may have caused it. I started Googling things like 'bacon and colitis' and other ridiculous things in a panic to try to find out how I managed to ruin my health, which up until that point was in a great state of remission. I then began to read forums about people who had been healthy and well and in total remission for 10 years or more who were suddenly struck down with a strong flare-up and ended up ill again for months or longer. It is strange, but even writing this now I start to feel small twinges in my stomach and I start to worry it may be coming back. I called my doctor first thing the next morning and was given a course of steroids again. It didn't really work. And I think this is the first time I ever really began to appreciate how bad the negative effects of the steroids really were. When I had taken them in the past I had always got an increased appetite and put on a little weight, but nothing like I experienced this time. It was making me so hungry that no matter what I ate I was never really satisfied. And everything I did eat just seemed to sit and build up in fat around my stomach and chest area. This was later then followed by my face, which I quickly realised was where the term 'moon face' came from.

The Prednisone steroid causes a redistribution of fat deposits in some people. Unfortunately for me it was around my lower belly and chest area, or 'moobs' as I called it, which had quickly built up enough fat that I could refer to them as man boobs. My face had also started getting rounder and filled out, with a sort of 'chubby cheek' appearance. As if the colitis symptoms were not making me feel down enough, I now had to deal with getting fat too. To be honest, although it did really depress me I can imagine it being a lot worse for a woman, especially those who don't have great metabolisms anyway. I know quite a few people who took Prednisone for different reasons and have had to come off it because it made them so fat and they just couldn't handle it. For me the thought of getting heavily bogged down with a colitis flare-up was far worse than any moon face or moob problem could give me so I carried on as planned. Unfortunately the treatment didn't really work. I got to the end of my course and I was as bad as I had ever been.

I managed to arrange an appointment with my specialist and I went to see him. For some reason that magical disappearing symptoms thing happened to me again. My belly had been bloated and sore for well over a month at this point and literally the moment I stepped foot into the specialist's room it went away. I explained the situation and he suggested that I increase my immunosuppressant dose. I was currently on a moderate to high dose anyway, but we would try the maximum and see how it went. We did discuss some other options if it didn't get any better, one of which was a new biological drug that had been approved to be used and another was surgery. The thought of surgery used to give me nightmares. There are many different types for people who suffer from colitis or similar conditions, but for me it basically involved cutting away part of the colon and having it redirected to the outside of the stomach where it would be fed into a colostomy bag. I can't really explain the reasons why, but for me this option was so low on the list that even in a life or death situation I would have to take time considering it. I had always imagined these bags were a thing for old people in nursing homes or hospitals, not active fit people in their late twenties. I suppose if I am being completely honest there is also a big element of embarrassment. If people see it or if I have to tell people I have one. I feel I would be even less inclined to go out and socialise than what I was at the peak of a flare-up.

I know there will be people reading this who believe it's stupid to think like that and it's probably true. It is just something I really struggled to come to terms with as a potential option and I still do. Anyway, I left and headed home. I immediately started on the increased dose and can you guess what else? Another course of steroids. By this point my belly fat and moobs were in full swing. Sometimes I looked in the mirror and I swear the mix of bloating and fat build up from the steroids made me look pregnant. I mean full-on, ready to pop nine months pregnant. I actually had to buy some new shirts because I was bursting out of most of the ones in my wardrobe. The one positive I took from being ill again was that my company agreed for me to go back to working in the office instead of offshore, at least until things settled down and my condition was under control. I knew the increased dose could take anywhere from three to six months to begin working again, which was a bit stressful, however luckily for me the newest course of steroids I started had dimmed the symptoms enough to make it bearable and allow me to go to work. I decided I was going to make use of this time to reinvestigate all the other potential treatments and cures I had researched previously.

FIVE

Meditate to Medicate

I have always had an interest in alternative therapies, especially things like massage and yoga and meditation techniques. There is a certain feeling of relief or relaxation you get from them that you can't get from anything else. I also knew from previous experience just how important your diet can be in relation to how you look and feel. The old 'You are what you eat' saying springs to mind. Exercise of course was another example of something non-medical that made me feel good and helped me to heal. Although I can't honestly say it had any positive effect on my colitis, or maybe it did and I just don't know it. I would say at the extreme peak of my flare-ups, I could not see how things could get any worse than they were. So I began researching everything I could find on the internet about 'cures for colitis' and 'unmedicated IBD treatment'. If you have suffered from this or something similar I have no doubt in my mind that these will have been in your search history at some point too. It is only natural to want to do so.

So the first treatment or supposed cure I came across that took my interest was an organic diet accompanied by some special supplements. A friend of mine who is obsessed with health and the use of organic food sent me a link to a website that focused on the treatment of many chronic diseases through diet. I contacted the owner of the company and explained my situation. He responded quite quickly with an email, which I am pretty sure was a copy and paste reply, telling me of how he has had many clients with colitis and Crohn's disease who are all in remission. Now although a large part of me knew this was too good to be true, when you're in times of desperation and need help you are willing to try anything. So in the email he advised me to try a few different things. The first was vitamin D3, which I had never heard of. It has some role in the immune system and cell repair. On paper that sounded great for what I was going through.

The next tip was to optimise my iodine concentration, which apparently much of the Western population is deficient in. The last was to do with food and diet. He advised me to cut out sugar, caffeine, flour and any grains. Now on this one I can partly agree with him. In fact this is one recommendation that kind of got me interested. The reason being that over the last few years there were certain things that I knew would trigger my symptoms. One of which was a high dose of caffeine, although somehow now I managed this without problems. Another consideration is sugar. Even now whenever I eat a lot of sugar in the form of cakes or chocolate or sweets, my stomach gets sore and bloated. Which is probably why I maybe struggled with my colitis more than others because I do have a very sweet tooth. Sometimes I just decide to eat chocolate and accept the consequences, which I know is probably the wrong thing to do. Anyway, the owner of the website provided me with a link to certain products, as well as a link to some of his client's success stories. When I watched them I wasn't entirely convinced by their testimonials. I decided to find the supplements elsewhere online and got them for a fraction of the price. I ordered them and started taking it straight away. I can't say if they were doing me any harm, in fact I am sure they weren't, but they certainly were not improving my colitis symptoms, at least not that I was aware of. I persevered with it for about three weeks, including the diet he had suggested, and I was none the better for it. I decided to give up and move on to something else.

The next treatment was a juicing diet. This actually worked, but it was unsustainable and I feel that it is actually a false cure and quite misleading. The way it worked (or at least how it was explained to me) was a means of giving your colon a break. No solid foods, no sugary processed junk, just pure organic vegetables juiced. It was claimed it would help you lose weight and also reduce or completely eradicate colitis. So I decided to try it out. Almost instantly I started to feel better. The juices basically consisted of celery and cabbage and one or two other things. That and water was all you could have. I think by day two my colitis symptoms were almost gone. No bloating, almost no blood at all, not very many urges to go to the toilet. I was also losing lots of weight, which to be honest wasn't a surprise when I was only taking in something like 800 calories a day. I think it was after day three or four when you were allowed some white fish, but this was still not enough. I got to day seven and gave up. I was weak, tired and absolutely starving. I was also struggling to sleep. When I really sat and thought about it and all the people's testimonials I had watched on YouTube and read about online, the idea of juicing to heal your colitis is slightly misleading. I mean I can't deny it certainly reduced my symptoms, but that is always going to be the case if you aren't putting any real food in your body. If there is no food travelling through my colon, there is nothing to irritate or worsen the inflammation. So in that sense it does work, but it doesn't heal or cure the disease. It just stops you experiencing the symptoms and in a very unsustainable way. I don't believe it is healthy or good for you to do that long term and in my honest opinion, whether it had been a week or a month or a year when I gave up, I genuinely feel the reintroduction of solid foods would just put me right back to where I started. So it was on to the next one.

I used to read a lot about self-healing, especially around meditation and yoga. After trying the supplements and juicing diet I was looking for something non-diet related. This seemed ideal. A lot of people, especially in the Far East, believe that the body has the ability to heal itself of anything, which in a lot of ways it does, but was colitis one of them? I thought probably not but I decided to give it a go anyway. I signed up to a yoga class not far from my office and also downloaded an app for my phone that gave me guided meditation sessions I could follow at home. There is a lot of evidence to suggest stress can be a major factor in managing a chronic condition, maybe not so much the root cause of colitis or Crohn's, but certainly in the trigger or flare-up of the condition. Yoga and meditation focused on reducing stress and helping you to manage them better, which in theory would reduce the probability of a flare-up happening or at least the severity of it. I was a bit doubtful, but I remained as positive as possible. Strangely enough, after my first session at the class there was an instant improvement of my condition so I decided to keep it up and I continued to go at least once a week every week, including a bit of meditation every day or when I could manage it. If I'm honest, on the whole looking back now I think it only really improved my symptoms around the time I was attending. If I went to class on a Thursday, by the time the weekend came around my condition would be as bad as it ever was. It could even happen sometimes as early as an hour or two after the session, depending on what was going on or what I had eaten. So in times of a flare-up, it is definitely a great tool to help, but in terms of remission or 'curing' it didn't work.

Another option I tried was the anti-inflammatory drugs I had been taking, but instead of oral tablets they were in a suppository form. These were absolutely horrendous and it blows my mind how anyone can ever manage them on a regular basis. It was basically a small tablet that you were meant to place inside your rectum in the evening before bed. However, the sensation of putting it in – never mind keeping it in – was just way too much for me. I couldn't even lie still, let alone relax and go to sleep with it in situ. I then switched it to an enema form. It came in a small plastic juice carton and had a plastic straw-like implement on the end. The idea was to squirt the fluid up inside you and it would coat the inside of the inflamed area and calm it down. This was also a huge fail. The biggest problem with it was that when you squirted it, you were also pressing air up, which then inflated you and made you need to pass wind, which in turn would push all the liquid back out again. I think during my worst days I did persevere with this for a while, but I genuinely don't think it was doing me any good. In fact in some way I think it almost accelerated the bloating symptoms or triggered them to get worse. Plus lying on my side naked on the cold bathroom tiles, trying to insert a big plastic tube up my bum isn't exactly the way I would like to be spending my evenings. Another one worth mentioning, although I never actually got around to trying it due to the fact it wasn't available in the UK and sounds a bit weird, is faecal transplant, also known as faecal bacteriotherapy. It is the process of restoring the bacteria with an infusion of faeces from a donor. It is basically taking stool samples of someone with a healthy colon and placing them inside the colon of someone with colitis. I think, although I'm not completely sure, it replaces the missing or damaged bacteria with new healthy functioning bacteria. I remember when I was researching it hadn't been approved for use, but I think elsewhere in Europe you could go and get it done. It sounds a bit disgusting, but if there was even a tiny whisper of hope it would work, then it would be worth it.

I am sure there are many more alternative treatments or reported cures, but these are all I really read about or tried. However, I would like to think in the near future we will have a definitive answer on what triggers colitis flare-ups and how to treat or even possibly cure them completely.

SIX

———

Vacant or Occupied?

As I have already mentioned, one of the biggest problems with colitis is not the pain or the blood or the bloating or all the tablets and other medication you need to get through. It really is just the frequent and overwhelming urge to find a toilet in a very small amount of time. I can remember when I was young I would go to the bathroom for a bowel movement once a day and it was almost like clockwork. Once a day at the same time without a single problem. And if for any reason I couldn't go then I would just wait until later in the day. I am aware this is the case for most people and I really miss those times. I didn't realise until I got ill just how much of a luxury that truly is. The amount of 'close calls' I have had since suffering from colitis over the last few years is ridiculous. When growing up I could never use a public toilet or even a school toilet for that matter. The thought of trying to do a 'number two' anywhere but the comfort of my own home was just completely out of the question. Then as time went on and my colitis got worse I was forced to learn to go wherever was available. I started building up a certain tolerance to what I deemed to be an adequate toilet facility, because quite frankly most of the time I didn't have a choice. I can remember this one time I was in a bar during the day having lunch. It was a sunny afternoon and it was quite busy. It may have been a Sunday on a bank holiday weekend, but I can't remember. I wasn't even drinking, I had been on freshly squeezed orange juice and lemonade. I had finished my meal and was sitting chatting when all of a sudden my stomach distended. I sat for a moment and it went away. I knew I was going to be heading home within the next 10 minutes and decided to try to wait it out, which when you have colitis very rarely works for you. At that point an old school friend came into the bar who I hadn't seen for years and I felt obliged to stand with him and catch up. The whole time we were talking my stomach was churning and I was trying to wait for a polite gap in the conversation to get myself away. Around 15 minutes later he was still asking questions. My stomach felt like it was about to explode and I was already 99% sure I wasn't going to make it to the toilet anyway. The conversation ended and I turned and headed straight for the stairs up to the bathroom. When I got there the first two doors I tried had 'occupied' on the handle and they were locked, which was my worst nightmare. I grabbed the third door and to my relief it swung open. I had no time to check what I was doing and I just sat down and literally exploded into the toilet with mostly air as well as some blood. At least I had made it and the panic was over. Then I looked down and realised the toilet seat had been urinated on and there was even hair on it that then stuck to my leg as I stood up. It was disgusting. At least there was toilet roll, I thought to myself – always look on the bright side.

I think after that I really did start planning my days around where there were toilets situated and even started judging bars and restaurants on how good their facilities were rather than the food, drink and atmosphere. It's something you never really take notice of when you're perfectly healthy, but it really makes a difference when you aren't. I found myself avoiding certain events or even meeting at one place and then going home when everyone moved to the next venue purely on whether or not there was a toilet available... or should I say an adequate toilet. I hadn't taken much notice before but the amount of bars and restaurants and especially nightclubs that don't have locks on toilet doors or even have basic things like toilet roll is astonishing. I have lost count the amount of times I have had to hold doors closed with my hands or feet while sat on the toilet. Not to mention having to wait until the room is empty and penguin-walk through into the next cubicle looking for toilet roll. Sometimes though, however careful you are you are always going to find yourself in a position when you are stuck or have nowhere to go.

I remember a particularly significant time when I

was travelling from Aberdeen down to Glasgow. I was driving down the motorway and was just over halfway through my journey. I stopped by a McDonald's drive-through and ordered a cheeseburger and fries as well as a milkshake. It was not long after I had eaten this that I realised it was not agreeing with my stomach at all. It began cramping up and I knew it wasn't going to be long before I had to pull over. I passed a sign that said services in five miles. There was absolutely no way I was managing that. The cramps became frequent and severe. I made the decision that I was going to pull over on the next available layby. When I did there were two other cars in front of me. Two guys got out and started climbing their way onto the grass verge. They were both chatting to each other while doing a wee, so I assume they must have been friends or colleagues. I desperately wanted them to hurry up because obviously I was desperate for you-know-what, which is bad enough at the side of the road as it is without two other people being there as well. Unfortunately I couldn't hold it in. It was to go on the grass in front of them or do it in my car. I chose the grass. I quickly jumped out of the car and ran up the verge. By the time I did both guys were already unzipped and facing the fence, chatting away to each other as they did. I got up to the fence and moved as far along as I could beside a large wooded area, although in reality I was still only a few metres away from them. Sure enough one of the guys must have noticed me out of the corner of his eye. He glanced over briefly and kind of gestured forward saying, "it's got to be done – when you need to go, you need to go." I nervously laughed and nodded with agreement before proceeding to pull my jeans down and squat behind a bush. The look on this guy's face was absolutely priceless and to be honest his embarrassment and his clear feeling of not knowing where to look actually made me feel a whole lot better about the situation. I don't know if it was the relief of the immediate symptoms or the way the two men awkwardly scrambled back down the verge and into their car as quickly as they could, but I actually laughed out loud. It was one of those moments in life where you sort of just go, oh well – it's done now.

SEVEN

Remission is the Mission

I think it was around the fourth- or fifth-month point into the increased dosage of the immunosuppressant that I started to feel better. I was no longer taking steroids and my weight had levelled out again. My work improved and so did my social life. Most importantly I was able to get back into fitness and found my way into a regular gym routine very quickly. This is something that I feel really helped not only improve my symptoms, but has and continues to have a real impact on maintaining my remission. It's something I think is worth mentioning to tell you about what I do and don't do to ensure my colitis symptoms stay at bay. I know everyone is different and it is an extremely complicated disease, but I want to write down everything I know that has a positive effect on me and hopefully if you are a sufferer from colitis or Crohn's, it can help you too.

The first thing is spicy food. I am not one for particularly hot food anyway, but when I do have something with a bit of spice, it certainly does wreak havoc on my stomach. Whenever I eat Indian food, such as curries or spiced meat, my stomach bloats and although there isn't much pain at the time I usually feel it more the next day. It is a sort of uncomfortable feeling within my stomach and no matter what I do it doesn't go away. I don't know for a fact if it is the spice itself I'm reacting to or something that goes into the sauce or marinade, but I try my best to avoid it anyway.

The next is alcohol. I have gone through phases thinking some types of alcohol were better than others. In fact for a long time I believed that it was just beer that made me ill and the rest was fine. To a certain extent that's true, but if I am being honest and really thinking about it, I never really feel particularly well after any alcohol. Not in the sense of a hangover, but in the sense of my stomach bloating or an increased frequency in my urge to go to the toilet. When I do go out these days I stick to wine or spirits, because beer definitely has a negative effect on me. I would say within about two mouthfuls of a fizzy ale or lager my stomach starts to go hard and sore and I need the toilet.

This brings me onto my next point, which I think could be linked due to the bubbles in carbonated beverages. Fizzy drinks. I have always been a fan of fizzy drinks such as Coke or Fanta, and of course being Scottish my favourite: Irn-Bru. However, I know now this has an adverse effect on my symptoms. I thought for a while it was something to do with the amount of sugar in it and I then switched to the diet or zero versions, which for some time seemed to help. I then thought it may have been the caffeine that was upsetting me so I tried a non-caffeinated, no sugar version and I was reasonably fine, but in all honesty I didn't enjoy drinking it. So now I do still indulge in sugar-free fizzy drinks now and again, but I try to limit how much I have, or as with other things just enjoy it and accept the consequences.

Sugar is another thing on this list. Although I have mentioned it earlier, I think I need to mention it again. Sweets, chocolate, cake, biscuits and so on – all of these things have a really negative effect on my colitis. For me this was one of the biggest problems. I have such a sweet tooth. Something I didn't know before I got colitis is that sugar is an inflammatory. So the more we eat, the more our body will become inflamed and in regular large doses it can cause low-grade chronic inflammation. So as you probably know by now, colitis is the inflammation of the colon and the immunosuppressant tablets are designed to reduce that inflammation, which when you eat sugar is working against that. For a while I tried to cut sugar out of my diet completely, but after some time I realised that you have got to have a bit of give and take. That doesn't mean you can start binging on sweets, but having something sugary now and again in moderation is completely fine in both my opinion and experience. I suppose you just have to listen to your own body and decide what you can handle.

Now without a doubt caffeine is a huge trigger for me. Not necessarily a flare-up trigger, but it certainly initiates the same symptoms: an urge or need to go to the toilet, especially after a large meal. I remember once I was visiting my parents and I received a call from someone at work. I think it was one of my managers, although I can't remember the details I recall it being really important. After a few minutes my father had come into the room and handed me a small cup of coffee. He had just returned from a trip in Italy and had brought back some coffee beans and espresso cups. I didn't think much of it and continued to sip away on this freshly made Italian espresso. Within about a minute, my stomach just locked up. I can remember pacing round in circles in the room trying to maintain a normal level of conversation on the call, wishing for it to end. Although he continued to speak I couldn't find the correct moment to excuse myself from the call. He just kept talking and talking and my stomach felt like it just kept getting bigger and bigger at each passing second. It got to the point where I couldn't hold it in any longer and I ran to the toilet, phone clamped to my ear, in the hope that I might be able to relieve the pressure silently. I sat down, trying my best to be as quiet as I could, but as soon as I did air and blood just exploded out of me so loud it echoed around the bathroom. My manager stopped instantly mid-speech and I knew he must have heard it. I panicked, ended the call abruptly and turned my phone off. I waited until I was finished and turned it on again. I called him back apologising saying my phone had run out of battery. He sounded a bit off with me and I'm pretty sure he knew exactly what he had heard, but it was never spoken of again.

I mentioned earlier about protein supplements and I think it is important I speak about this in more detail. When I first went into remission from colitis I was practically living off of protein shakes and protein bars. I think I sort of ignored the symptoms at the time for some reason, but now on reflection I think there was very rarely ever a time when I would drink a shake and my stomach didn't get sore and inevitably result in a mild colitis flare-up. I don't believe there is a great deal of research to suggest exactly why they are bad for you, but the moment I go near even just a spoonful of a synthetic protein, like powder for shakes, bars, pancakes or whatever the product, I get really ill. The symptoms are very like colitis and I have friends who also have experienced this, even though they don't have bowel or colon issues. My recommendation is if even if you are slightly unsure, just avoid them and stick to wholesome natural foods where possible.

The last and I think most commonly experienced among most colitis and Crohn's sufferers I have spoken with is stress. To my mind it really is what initiated my colitis in the first place and definitely has a major impact on when I get flare-ups. I remember when I was at my doctor discussing my symptoms and I said that I thought stress was having an impact on me. He asked what I was stressed about. I thought for a moment and I replied, "I don't know, everything I suppose." He gave me a funny look. The problem was that I couldn't really pinpoint anything in particular. I have been someone who has always suffered periods of stress and anxiety throughout my life. I am quite bad at worrying about things and then over-analysing every detail or possible outcome. Although there was no particular incident in my case, I think general life stresses such as exams, job interviews, relationship break-ups, family problems and money or career worries can all be enough to trigger a flare-up. The problem is there's no quick fix for reducing these everyday stresses. It is more about learning to manage them and not allowing it to affect your condition. My problem was the symptoms of the colitis were giving me high levels of stress, which in turn caused my colitis to get worse, which then made me more stressed. It was a never-ending cycle. What I decided to do was to try meditation and yoga, as mentioned earlier, which certainly helped even if it was in the short term. Another thing I tried was hypnotherapy. Although I didn't use it as a treatment for my colitis, I wanted to try to see if it could reduce my stress levels and hopefully in turn reduce my colitis. Funnily enough, it did work reasonably well. Although I would say it was quite a short-term fix, it was enough to reduce the general symptoms and diminish the stress cycle. I also believe using this periodically, even when in remission, can help ensure you stay healthy and symptom-free going forwards.

EIGHT

More than Meets the Eye

I can recall one point where I had been off work due to a flare-up and I hadn't left the house in a couple of days. A friend of mine asked if I would like to go for lunch and I decided to take him up on the offer. I thought the fresh air might help. While we were sitting at the table a colleague of mine came into the café we were in. He walked right up to me and one of the first things he said was, "I thought you were off sick?" I told him he was right and that I was unwell and he kind of laughed as if I was joking. I realised at that point how little people understand – not only about colitis, but about health and sickness in general. I felt these external pressures quite regularly throughout the years suffering from the condition – the symptoms were not obvious but I was in a bad way, but no one could tell by looking at me. Another time I remember clearly when I was at the tail-end of one of my worst flare-ups I had managed to get myself to the gym after almost a week of being stuck at home. One of the most overlooked tools for general health and well-being is exercise. I was advised by so many people and read about so many proven reasons why exercise is important in achieving and maintaining remission from colitis. However, to the outside world this can be something that's hard to understand. When someone sees you at a gym or out running somewhere when you are meant to be off work due to sickness, they see it as some sort of sign that you are faking it. I had only just stepped on the treadmill and began a light jog when two people who worked in my office walked in. They approached me at the side of the treadmill and asked how I was doing. I said I was okay, because in reality at that exact moment in time I *was* okay even though for the last seven days I really hadn't been. One then suggested I should be going back to work, which I replied that I wasn't ready for yet. He then gestured towards the treadmill as if to say, well what are you doing here then? As if only healthy and fit people can come to the gym. I didn't respond. It quickly became apparent to me that he must have told a few people I had been in the gym and was getting on fine because within around two days I had a call from someone at work asking me to come to the office. It wasn't the easiest of phone calls and it really stressed me out. The thought of being there in the condition I was in and how I was feeling was a horrible thought. I could tell by the voice on the end of the phone that they thought I was lying and they then suggested I go to see the company doctor for a second opinion.

I have actually lost count the amount of times people who are close to me have judged or made assumptions on how I am 'really' feeling. Like whether or not I am faking it or over-exaggerating my symptoms. I mean, if you were able to go to the gym today how can you not come on a night out? Or if you went out for lunch this afternoon, why can't you come to the party tonight? I wonder if they would be making this call if I had a cast around my leg or were walking with crutches. Would they have the same attitude if I had bandages around my head with blood or scars on my skin? I think probably not. People only like to believe what they can see and to be perfectly honest up until I had colitis I would have probably been the same.

Although I would never wish this on anyone, now that I am healthy again I can honestly say that it has done so much for me as a person. It has changed me dramatically and completely reinvented how I look at the world. It has given me the ability to understand that everyone you meet – regardless of age, appearance or background – have all walked a journey to get to where they are and you never really know what is going on with someone. It has also taught me how people react to things differently. I remember meeting someone who had been diagnosed quite recently with colitis and them telling me how much it had affected their life. They got really upset recounting it all and I tried my best to make them feel comfortable about it. After chatting for a while I came to realise that their condition was, in the grand scheme of IBD as a whole, extremely mild. In fact they rarely took medication and it only bothered them every now and then. I came away from the conversation thinking about how lucky they were and how badly I wanted to be in their position, whereas they had spent the whole time telling me how unlucky they felt and how much it had ruined their day-to-day life. On the flip side to that, I've met people who have probably been envious of my condition. People who have tried every medication known to science, and it either hasn't worked or has made them feel worse. People who have then had to go on to have surgery or multiple operations in an attempt to just live a normal life or stay alive at a bare minimum. When I think back, although I had lost friends, a partner, career opportunities and I had gone through quite a lot of mental and physical pain, it really wasn't that bad.

So here I am two years later and I can honestly say I am feeling great. I am in complete remission from the symptoms and I have started to rebuild myself into a normal life again. I have possibly had one or two odd days where I felt it may have been an attack coming on, but on the whole I've felt good. I suppose you never really know what will happen next, but this is the longest period I have felt well in almost 10 years and I genuinely believe it is here to stay. It's weird – even when I write the words '10 years' it doesn't seem real. It is as if it was a nightmare and I have finally woken up. A lot of the dark times seem a blur to me now and when I try to think back to exactly how I was feeling or what was going through my mind it's as if it never happened.

When I was growing up I could never have envisioned my life to be the way it is now. Neither could I ever have ever imagined myself being diagnosed with a serious chronic disease. It was only when I began to suffer that I learnt the importance of health and the unimportance of material things. The want for fancy clothes and new trainers, big biceps and a six pack, cars and holidays or attention and respect from people who didn't really matter was gone for ever. I learned to want for basic things like the ability to go to work, a loving family, genuine reliable friends, a roof over my head, clothes on my back regardless of the label and most importantly the ability to wake up every morning and embrace life to the fullest.

It was during my worst flare-ups I would watch people go through life without a care in the world, happily floating along. I would become jealous and wish I could be in that place. But I slowly began to realise that what was happening to me wasn't just a painful negative experience. It was an awakening to a world that I had been surrounded by my whole life, but I had never really seen it. I discovered suffering in people close to me that I had never acknowledged before. I found respect for people for enduring things that I had never properly considered. I saw great strength in people who suffered in silence and still maintained a normal life. I felt courage from people that were invisible to me before.

By no means do I believe this journey is over, but I feel the road behind me was the most difficult I have had to walk. I believe now if it gets tough again I have the experience and tools to get through it. In the same way, I also believe you can. If you are someone who suffers from colitis or Crohn's or some other chronic condition, then I want you to know whether it's getting caught short in a public place, the side of the motorway or just three metres from your own bathroom. Whether it's getting raised eyebrows and curious looks from all those people around you who just don't understand. Whether it's those sleepless nights or restless days sapping your energy. Whether it's the bloating, cramps and blood keeping you glued to a toilet for days on end. Whether it's that overwhelming fear that it's getting worse and developing into something more serious. Whether it's the cold realisation your social life now revolves around access to a decent bathroom. And most specifically when you feel so down and depressed that you believe you have nothing left... There is light at the end of the tunnel. Believe me. And just remember, as you go through life every single person you meet has a past. Every single person you meet is on a journey. Never judge someone on how they appear to you.

There is always more than meets the eye.

EPILOGUE

Sometimes during some of my flare-ups, especially the really bad ones where I couldn't even leave the house, I really did feel like my life was over. It was mostly career-based worries or fears about losing things I enjoyed that affected me the most. I did question on a daily basis whether or not I was going to have to completely reinvent myself. The stress this adds to your body, which is already at or beyond its limits, is something that you definitely don't need more of. So I have decided to make a list of some notable people over recent times who have had some form of IBD and the things they have achieved while suffering or came back to achieve upon regaining health, some of which include performing at the highest of levels in politics, sports and entertainment.

John F. Kennedy, the 35th president of America. Well known for his assassination in 1963, however unknown to most for being a long-time sufferer of stomach problems, which were later suspected to be the result of ulcerative colitis. This was hidden from the public during his presidency but it is something he struggled with most of his life, which began when he was a child.

Dwight D. Eisenhower, the 34th president of America, was diagnosed with Crohn's in 1956 and consequently went on to have surgery.

Shinzō Abe, the prime minister of Japan. He suffered from ulcerative colitis that later led to his resignation in 2007. In an interview with the Australian TV network ABC in 2008 he said, "I would need to go to the lavatory 30 times a day. It would be absolutely impossible to perform the heavy duties of the prime minister." However upon moving on to a new medication, he was soon not only able to control his condition, but then went on to return to his role as prime minister a few years later and is still doing so now.

Gregory Itzin, Emmy nominated American film and television actor, best known for his role in crime drama 24. During the filming of the show his UC had got so bad that he ended up in hospital. However, he then returned to play a role in more movies and television shows, including being nominated and winning awards for doing so.

Sunny Anderson, a celebrity chef who has been living with UC for over 20 years, not only continues to do so at a high level, but has also launched a website designed to educate those who IBD about the role of diet and nutrition in managing symptoms.

Dan Reynolds, the lead singer of Imagine Dragons, announced that he had UC and another related disease called ankylosing spondylitis, which causes the spine and other areas of the body to become inflamed. After being able to manage the diseases, he still continues to make music.

Sir Steve Redgrave, a British rower who won gold in five consecutive Olympics, speaks openly about the struggles of living with UC. He is now a supporter for Crohn's and Colitis UK.

Amy Brenneman, well-known Hollywood actress particularly for her roles in Judging Amy and Grey Anatomy, is a long-time sufferer of UC.

Kathleen Baker, an American competition swimmer who specialises in the freestyle and backstroke events. She was diagnosed with Crohn's when she was 11 years old. She was told her dreams of becoming an Olympian were over. She then went on to win a gold and silver medal in the 2016 Summer Olympics.

Rolf Benirschke, an American football player, was struck down with UC in the second season of his career. He then went onto have major surgery that nearly cost him his life. However he came back with a successful career spanning 10 years and was the third most accurate placekicker in history at the time of his retirement in 1987.

This list could go on, but I think it gets across the point that I'm making. It has been demonstrated that if these people can come back from ill health and not only continue a life and survive, but actually perform and compete at the highest of levels, then you can too.

Some links to websites and forums which you may find useful.

https://www.crohnsandcolitis.org.uk/
https://www.crohnscolitisfoundation.org/
https://www.crohnscolitiscommunity.org/crohns-colitis-forum
https://www.facebook.com/crohnsandcolitisuk/
https://www.facebook.com/groups/CCUKforum/
https://www.facebook.com/ccfafb/

ACKNOWLEDGMENTS

———————

I want to firstly say a big thank you to anyone who's taken time out of their day to read this book. Knowing that even just one person may find some comfort or positive energy in the experiences I have shared is such a wonderful thought. I also want to say thank you to all the doctors, nurses, friends and family who have supported my journey along the way. I truly could not have got through it all if it wasn't for you.

Finally, I want to say a big thank you to all my fellow IBD sufferers for your continued efforts in fighting every day and never giving up. Each and every day we come together and open up about our struggles is each day we grow stronger.

Thank you.

Printed in Great Britain
by Amazon

59121881R00052